YOUR KNOWLEDGE HAS VALUE

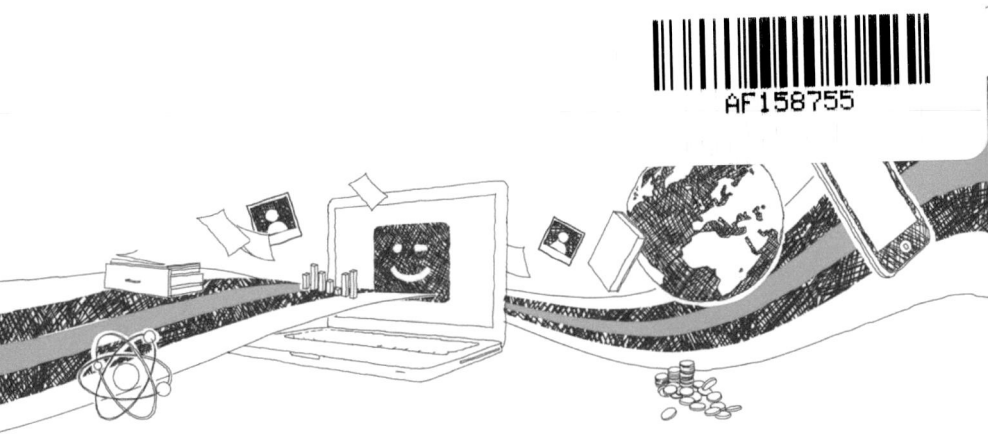

- We will publish your bachelor's and master's thesis, essays and papers

- Your own eBook and book - sold worldwide in all relevant shops

- Earn money with each sale

Upload your text at www.GRIN.com
and publish for free

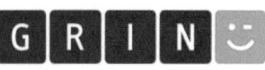

Bibliographic information published by the German National Library:

The German National Library lists this publication in the National Bibliography; detailed bibliographic data are available on the Internet at http://dnb.dnb.de .

This book is copyright material and must not be copied, reproduced, transferred, distributed, leased, licensed or publicly performed or used in any way except as specifically permitted in writing by the publishers, as allowed under the terms and conditions under which it was purchased or as strictly permitted by applicable copyright law. Any unauthorized distribution or use of this text may be a direct infringement of the author s and publisher s rights and those responsible may be liable in law accordingly.

Imprint:

Copyright © 2016 GRIN Verlag, Open Publishing GmbH
Print and binding: Books on Demand GmbH, Norderstedt Germany
ISBN: 9783668540705

This book at GRIN:

http://www.grin.com/en/e-book/373961/aged-care-physiotherapy-are-we-doing-it-right

Nitiish Matthew

Aged care Physiotherapy. Are we doing it right?

GRIN Publishing

GRIN - Your knowledge has value

Since its foundation in 1998, GRIN has specialized in publishing academic texts by students, college teachers and other academics as e-book and printed book. The website www.grin.com is an ideal platform for presenting term papers, final papers, scientific essays, dissertations and specialist books.

Visit us on the internet:

http://www.grin.com/

http://www.facebook.com/grincom

http://www.twitter.com/grin_com

Table of Contents

- AGED CARE PHYSIOTHERAPY: ARE WE DOING IT RIGHT?... 1
- DUTIES OF AGED CARE PHYSIOTHERAPIST 2
- BARRIERS IN AGED CARE PHYSIOTHERAPY 3
- AGED CARE FUNDING INSTRUMENT 4
- PROS OF BEING AN AGED CARE PHYSIOTHERAPIST:... 6
- REFERENCES 8

AGED CARE PHYSIOTHERAPY: ARE WE DOING IT RIGHT?

As per the latest census in 2016, there are more than 3.2 million Australians between 65-84 years of age. There are 487,000 people aged over 85 years of age (AIHW, 2017). Over these years there have been tremendous growth in population and also a decrease in a number of deaths secondary to major conditions like cancer, COPD, CVD, etc. The Australian Bureau of statistics predicts the total number of Australians over the age of 65 years to increase more than 6 million by 2051. It is estimated that by 2051, around 3.5 million people in the older age group will be using aged care system (APA, 2012).

Negative effects of aging include changes observed in muscle strength, joint cartilage, bone density and body fat, which leads to poor fitness, thereby causing further health implications such as dyspnea, hypertension, arthritis, circulatory issues, stroke, etc. (Maguire, 2016). Another common health issue noticed in the aged population is the psychological disorders which affects cognition and orientation. Eg. Dementia, delirium.

Geriatric (Aged care) Physiotherapy was introduced as a specialty in Physiotherapy in 1989. Since then, Physiotherapists have worked together to find out and understand all the age related problems which could be treated through Physiotherapy. Physiotherapists play a major role as primary care practitioners in treating and managing the functional limitations in the older generation due to all the common conditions such as stroke, Parkinson's disease, arthritis, COPD, cancer and joint replacement surgeries. Physiotherapists check the suitability of particular modalities or interventions for the treatment of musculoskeletal, neurovascular and cardiopulmonary conditions. Their role is important in the rehabilitation after a fall, for injury prevention and also for functional incontinence (APA, 2012).

Benefits of geriatric physiotherapy in improving mobility and balance, strength, increasing confidence in performing activities of daily living and enabling an active life for more years, is proven worldwide.

DUTIES OF AGED CARE PHYSIOTHERAPIST

An aged care physiotherapist is like the jack of all trades. They should have sound knowledge of respiratory care, orthopedics, medicine and neurology, along with psychosocial aspects, to provide a holistic and client-centered care.

General principles practiced in aged care physiotherapy (Ramaswami, 2015):

- Find the root cause of disability, i.e the pathological cause/ injury, which makes the life of the clients dependent on others.
- Maintain the functioning of the body systems to its optimum level. It is the role of physiotherapist to help older people to use all the body systems fully to enhance mobility and independence.
- Enabling a pain-free and comfortable life to all clients.
- Health promotion by prevention of health problems for the future.

The therapist should focus on the patient's goals while planning a treatment protocol. At the same time, the treatment should be centered towards management and improvement of the health condition. Most of the time, it is difficult to manage and improve the health of the client completely. On these occasions, the Physiotherapist can focus towards the chief complaints of their client, thereby providing pain relief and care for them. It is not always possible to reverse the health problems of the clients and return them to earlier states of health, but the key is to help them function to the best of their ability.

It is a complex task to understand the problems of clients suffering from brain disorders such as dementia. People with dementia face difficulty in expressing the nature and site of pain. They show episodes of depression or agitation as a result of their health problems. Pain in these clients also affects cognition, concentration, and motivation to any therapeutic intervention (Chartered Society of Physiotherapy, 2017). Physiotherapists, with their effective communication skills and knowledge, can diagnose the sites of pain and provide appropriate management to improve the quality of living of these clients. They can provide proper family and carer education, to support and manage the lifestyle of aged people with dementia.

Falls are a common problem noticed in elderly people due to their neurological, skeletal and visual disorders (Bloodsmyth, 2016). A well-maintained exercise program can reduce the chances of falls in elderly by 54 percent (Falls Action, 2015). Therapists need to assess the root cause of each fall, which is either extrinsic or intrinsic and come up with appropriate solutions to prevent them in the future.

Hence, Geriatric Physiotherapists witness the signs and symptoms in patients, which are observed in other streams of Physiotherapy. An aged care Physiotherapist need to follow the same assessment and treatment protocol which they would use with other populations. But the main problem is that the elderly generation is unable to get access to regular physiotherapy in Australia. This is due to a number of reasons. The major reason is that there are only a small number of Physiotherapists willing to work in the aged care sector. The poor funding provided by Medicare and ACFI towards physiotherapy programs is another common barrier (APA, 2010). People living in rural areas also suffer a lot more because of the smaller number of centers providing physiotherapy, and other barriers such as access to transport, long distance, and disability (PCare, 2016).

BARRIERS IN AGED CARE PHYSIOTHERAPY

> Disinterest in Physiotherapists to work in Aged care sector:

- Physiotherapists feel that the workload in aged care is too much, stressful and boring.
- They feel there is less professional development in this field.
- Workload increases if the physiotherapy assistants have less knowledge and experience, thereby leading to decreased job satisfaction (Higgins, 2012).
- Salary is less compared to other streams of Physiotherapy.

> Government rules

- There is no national framework stating the amount of Physiotherapy care in terms of duration to be provided for the residents in aged care sector.

> Funds are inadequate:

- The major funding providers like Aged care funding instrument grant no funds for rehabilitation of functional independence, falls prevention, strength training.

- Medicare chronic disease management program gives the limitation to claim only 5 allied health services in one year, and this is decided by the general practitioner.
- The funding providers like Rural Health Workforce Australia, which used to allocate funds/reimbursements for therapists who shift to more rural areas, does not have such practices at present, due to a change in laws (MHC, 2016).

AGED CARE FUNDING INSTRUMENT

- It provides financial grants for treatment of residents in aged care homes. It focuses on passive pain management protocols and nothing for active functional training for independence.
- Physiotherapy treatments according to ACFI include pain management with the help of therapeutic massage or electrotherapeutic modalities, which could be given to the residents at least once or 4 times per week respectively. Duration is set at 20 minutes per session from 2017.
- Physiotherapists decide the frequency of treatments (once per week or 4 times per week) which should be then approved by ACFI.
- The present model is prescriptive, and not based on clinical assessments or need based, thus not evidence based to improve the quality of life of residents.

Many Physiotherapy organizations and Therapists have come forward with their views against the drawbacks of this tool. Rik Dawson, Gerontology chief, APA appreciates the focus on pain management in the funds allocated to residents but points out the failure in not including exercises or evidence-based practices like Cognitive behavior therapy, joint mobilization, postural correction, as part of pain management. He adds that the evidences of the benefits of exercises for older people with Arthritis are more than that for massage or TENS (Egan, 2016).

Jennifer Hewitt, APA member, adds that frequent falls inside aged care centers form a major factor in the increasing pain in the residents. The cost of the falls in these residents is more than 20% of the total falls of the healthcare system. Prevention of falls becomes a priority in these homes for maintaining the health of residents with regards to pain, independence and mobility. Hewitt proved the benefits of exercise over pain as well as prevention of falls.

Anita Powell, the executive office of ESSA, is disappointed that exercise physiology is not included in the ACFI tool, thus the aged care centers do not appoint an exercise physiologist. Apart from just mentioning about the strength and pain management benefits of exercise for the older population, she also pointed out the psychological benefits of exercises on these populations. She proved this by presenting the evidence of increased socialization seen in isolated residents, happiness and improvement in health status of residents, and also the interest and fun which the residents witness during group exercise programs (Australian Ageing Agenda, 2015).

At the same time, there have been public comments on media stating that ACFI allows unethical practices. Families of residents in nursing homes have reported their concern that aged care providers keep searching for ways to increase the funding, but there is still no evidence of relevant improved outcomes for the residents (Aged care crisis Inc., 2015).

APA has submitted a request to Government to reform the plan of ACFI, and allow the residents to benefit from Physiotherapy managed exercise while reducing pain as well as independence and quality of life (APA, 2010).

For these reasons, Physiotherapists in Australia refuse to work in aged care. To solve this problem, Australian employers hire a number of overseas physiotherapists on sponsorship work visas. In 2012, 3006 out of 17075 employed Physiotherapists were from countries other than Australia. The number of therapists hired on 457 sponsorship work visas increased from 90 in 2009 to 118 in 2013. Similarly, therapists hired through employer-sponsored permanent visas or general skilled migration visas are in high numbers each year (HWA, 2014). Physiotherapy has remained in skills shortage for many years, but a majority of the new therapists joining streams other than aged care, puts all the aged care residential and nursing homes in crisis. It is observed that Residential homes in Australia hire Physiotherapists part time: 1 day per week or on-call. The high number of fresh graduate physiotherapists (with nil relevant working experience) and occupation therapists working in the field of aged care is also due to the same reason of low number of Physiotherapists interested in this field.

PROS OF BEING AN AGED CARE PHYSIOTHERAPIST:

Compared to other streams of Physiotherapy, aged care has less challenges and workload. Despite the residents in residential and nursing homes having disorders and disabilities of various causes, the duty of Physiotherapist here is focused only on pain management as the key. In a nutshell, the basic duties expected by the aged care Physiotherapist in Australia are (W & L Aged care services, 2017):

- Pain management
- Reassessments to evaluate the outcome of interventions prescribed for residents
- Use of evidence-based assessment tools
- Maintaining records of the treatment hours for each resident
- Making sure that all residents have their pain management sessions claimed from Government.

For nursing homes which run on funding from the Government, as all the funding agencies pay only for pain management through massage or TENS, the role of the Physiotherapist is confined to this basic management. It is solely the decision of Physiotherapist whether to include exercise management as an addition in the pain management program. These exercises could be used as a treatment plan for improving the mobility, strength, balance and gait of the residents.

Hence, full-time Physiotherapists in aged care are given full freedom to schedule their management as required, provided they follow the basic guidelines provided by ACFI for pain management.

Another plus point of being an aged care Physiotherapist is the salary. The average salary is $92,181 annually, i.e $43/hour, which is 1.5 times more than the median wage of Australia. New graduates can earn around $65,000 and experienced workers over $129,000 (Neuvoo, 2017).

The increase in the number of the geriatric population has added to the working hours of Physiotherapist. Physiotherapists spend 46% of their time on pain management treatments, 25% on non- pain management treatments and 29% on documentation, as per the survey by Australian Physiotherapy Association (APA 2014).

Apart from all this, it is the Physiotherapist who can bring a smile on the residents who are suffering from pain and dependence in the aged care centers. Spending time with them, even for a friendly conversation for a few minutes makes a lot of difference in their lives. It brings a sense of trust in their mind, when they understand there is somebody to look after their health problems, that there is somebody to go to if they are in pain.

Hence, a therapist can just go to the aged care facility and treat the residents just for the pain through massage or else make it worthwhile by including group exercise programs, balance classes, games sessions, walks with residents, use of stationary bikes or Swiss balls. Many therapists who work full time in such facilities already practice the latter and continue living a healthy and happy work-life, thereby providing an active quality of life for the residents as well. A survey by APA shows that 60% of the Physiotherapists believe that the consultation and treatment time is not adequate. Physiotherapists have already joined hands all over Australia to increase the work hours.

There are 5710 aged care residential homes in Australia. The number of older population will continue to grow. In 2056, the proportion of older Australians is expected to increase up to 8.7 million. By 2096, there will be more than 12.8 million Australians aged 65 years and above (AIHW, 2017). Australians are living longer, medical standards are getting better and better, but are we really preserving and improving aging with medicines? Every field has recognized the value of Physiotherapy in the field of Geriatrics, but less people are available in Australia to support this ageing population. If spreading love and increasing smiles is your motto as a Physiotherapist, think again, these elderly champions are waiting for a guiding hand and a piece of motivation from you.

REFERENCES

Aged care crisis Inc., (2015, Oct 13). Aged Care finding Instrument (ACFI). Aged care crisis.com. Retrieved from Aged care crisis resources database.

Australian Ageing Agenda, (2015, Feb 12). Anew call for Allied health in aged care. Australian Ageing Agenda. Retrieved from Industry, Research, and clinical database.

Australian Institute of health and welfare. (2017). Australia's changing age and gender profile. Australia Government. Retrieved from www.aihw.org.au

Australian Physiotherapy Association. (2010, July). Submission to the caring for older Australians inquiry. Productivity Commission, (pp. 3-11).

Australian Physiotherapy Association. (2012, June). Supporting older Australians. Australian Physiotherapy Association, (pp.1-2). Retrieved from www.physiotherapy.asn.au

Australian Physiotherapy Association. (2014). ACFI Survey. Australian Physiotherapy Association, (pp. 6-14).

Blood-Smyth, J. (2016). Physiotherapy for the elderly: Local Physio. Retrieved from www.local-physio.co.uk

Chartered Society of Physiotherapy. (2017). Physiotherapy works: Dementia care: Dementia action alliance. UK: CSP

Egan, N. (2016, June 1). Call for ACFI overhaul to cover exercise therapy for pain management. Australian Ageing Agenda. Retrieved from Health and Medical industry database.

Falls Action. (2015). Minimizing Falls: Falls screen. Retrieved from www.falls.ie

Higgins, C. (2012). Physiotherapy Assistants and the APA. Australian Physiotherapy Association. Retrieved from www.physiotherapy.asn.au

Human Workforce Australia. (2014). Workforce inflows. Australia's health workforce series- Physiotherapists in focus, (pp. 30- 33)

Maguire, A. (2016). Physiotherapy for elderly patients; How it works: Ballsbridge Physiotherapy clinic. Retrieved from https://ballsbridgephysio.ie

My Health career. (2016, Dec 24). Addressing Physiotherapy workforce shortages in rural and remote Australia. My health career. Retrieved from www.myhealthcareer.com.au

Neuvoo. (n.d.). Aged care physiotherapist salary in Australia. Retrieved May, 2017 from https://au.neuvoo.com/salary/Aged-Care-Physiotherapist-salary

Physiotherapists Aged care, PCare, (2016). The growing rural population. Retrieved from www.pcare.com.au

Ramaswamy, B. (2015). Physiotherapy settings and onward referral: Physiotherapy and older people. Retrieved from physiopedia.

Wellness and Lifestyle Aged care services, (2017). 8 things your aged care Physiotherapist should be doing. Physiotherapy articles. Retrieved from www.wellnesslifestyles.com.au

YOUR KNOWLEDGE HAS VALUE

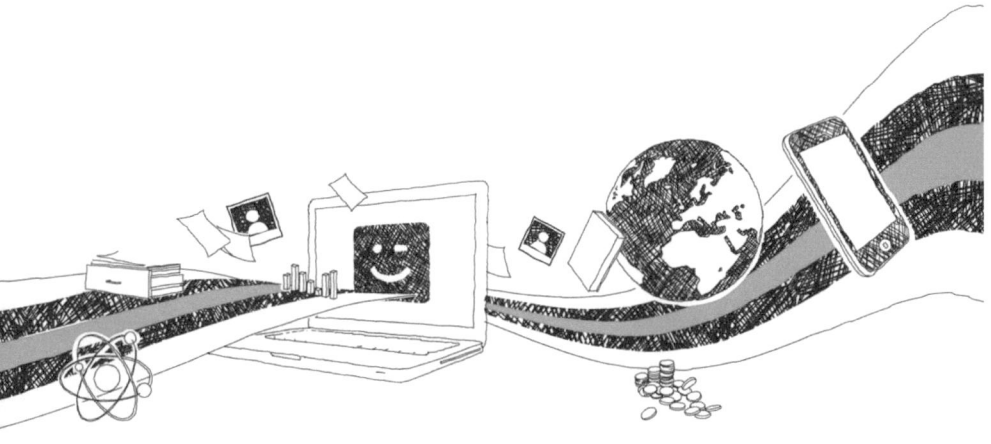

- We will publish your bachelor's and master's thesis, essays and papers

- Your own eBook and book - sold worldwide in all relevant shops

- Earn money with each sale

Upload your text at www.GRIN.com
and publish for free

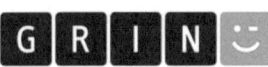